LOOKING

YOUNG

FOREVER

NATURAL ANTI AGING TIPS ON HOW TO LIVE FOREVER WITHOUT GETTING OLD

Dr. David A, Gundry.

Contents

INTRODUCTION

I don't think you should go out and buy anti-aging skincare right now but maintaining a certain lifestyle is definitely crucial in preventing signs of aging as always preventative methods are far better than reversing the damage.

So, today I'm going to teach you how to preserve the youth and maintain a certain lifestyle from diet to skin care habits to lifestyle habit. So how does our skin age? All living species including you and myself here are all programmed to die one day and sadly we are aging every single day and it's a natural process when it comes to skin aging.

There are three main things that are happening; one is the epidermis layer which is a surface layer of our skin. The skin renewal process slows down, therefore the useful and the younger looking skin is not really revealing itself anymore or it's much slower in the renewing process.

 Secondly is the dermis layer which is the lower level of the skin where it stores collagen elastin fiber which kind of makes up that elasticity, the firmness and the bounciness. It does break down by time and starts diminishing which results in fine lines wrinkles and skin sagginess.

 Lastly, there are lipids or our moisture barrier or our skin barrier that happens to break down by overtime by hormone levels and therefore your skin is becoming drier and drier as you age because your skin doesn't have that ability to protect the hydration to keep intact.

Now we're going to look into our diet first. If there is one thing that you take away from reading this book is to know that inflammation equals Pro aging.

CHAPTER ONE

WATCH WHAT YOU EAT AND DRINK

first of all let's stay away from all the inflammation causing foods such as sugar refined crabs, simple crab, alcohol industrial seed oils, red meat and processed foods and also there is a food processing or food group that you might want to stay away or pay more attention to called AG ease and that stands for advanced gyration end foods and this has more to do with the cooking method you choose to do than the actual ingredient or the food itself.

so by filling barbecuing, frying, roasting, baking and toasting will enhance inflammation causing a GE levels and certain foods such as animal fats and animal protein are more susceptible informing that a GE during this chemical processing.

A lot of studies do conclude that you should try more eschewing, boiling, steaming the food or consuming foods raw. I can suggest you to make some healthy switch in your current diet which I incorporate a lot; I see a huge difference in my body and in my skin as well.

 So I was switching white rice to brown rice, white bread to brown bread, red grilled or fried food to steamed and boiled food, conventional chips to something like healthy nuts, industrial seed oil to extra-virgin olive oil and minimize alcohol consumption to 1 glass of red win. (That is totally optional as well).

Now I want to introduce you to my five favorite anti-inflammatory foods that you can incorporate in a daily basis to fight against inflammation so you can balance all the processed food out.

First of all there's turmeric. Turmeric has a special compound called curcumin inside and that has a really free inflammatory effect. Turmeric is not my favorite taste so I like taking this as a tablet form and the product that I do take it with is available from herb. It's called fermented turmeric supplement and by a fermenting turmeric or any kind of food and naturally enhances the bioavailability which means that it's going to be absorbed way better in our system.

Secondly, we have garlic. Garlic is naturally anti-inflammatory, antifungal and antiviral and it's also known to boost your immune system as well, so I love putting sprinkling garlic powder in my avocados and in everything that I've cooked in my household.

 Thirdly, we have ginger. Ginger contains a compound called dangerous and that has a beautiful anti-inflammatory effect. Ginger also supports your digestive system as well, so if you ever feel constipated or bloated having a cup of ginger tea is highly recommended.

DARK LEAFY GREENS IN EVERY MEAL

We have dark leafy greens which are staple in my fridge every single day. In every meal I try to at least incorporate like a handful of dark leafy greens, they nourish our body at a cellular level and reduce overall inflammation. Another great anti-inflammatory food is actually cold water fish such as sardines and salmon.

 The second food group that you want to consume more is healthy fats, a lot of avocado, lot of chia seeds, and a lot of healthy nuts. This is such great news to me because I love these ingredients.

 Basically, your skin cells are comfortably wrapped around a fat layer or a fat cushion so once this gets depleted your skin will feel drier which can result in too much skin sagginess, more skin ageing.

A very crucial and essential fat soluble vitamin when it comes to overall skins health is vitamin A and we talked about a topical form of vitamin A which is basically retinol and retinol products but also internally you do want to consume a lot more vitamin A and rich foods vitamin E is another great fat cell of vitamin that you can consume for overall skins health. This helps to Preventing skins aging and essential fatty acids such as omega-3 is definitely beneficial for enhancing and plumping up and firming your skin.

 There is one supplement that I do take regularly for the past four to five years that takes up all the fatty acids and the fat soluble vitamins that you might need for your skin and that is now foods called " liver oil". This is a supplement that I started taking when I was researching about acne prone skin. It has a really high source of vitamin A and vitamin D and also omega-3 fatty acids. Omega-3 fatty acids will also lower the inflammation in your body.

 Third food group we want to incorporate more is definitely anti oxidant. I've been talking about the importance of antioxidants in the skincare in our food for the longest time but it is really crucial, especially if you are living in a city that's much polluted, that has a lot of environmental stressors or you are exposing yourself to a lot of UV rays. You need some antioxidants in your diet right now.

SOURCES OF ANTIOXIDANTS

 Dark chocolate has a lot of great fresh fruit berries and a lot of dark leafy green. You can choose green tea or matcha of your choice. If you are looking for some supplement options you can go for a coq10, resveratrol and also milk thistle.

 for me I just like packing everything in one powerful anti-aging smoothie and I will share my recipe right now. I love including at least one source of healthy fats whether that's avocado or chia seeds. In this case I'm going to reach for chia seeds if we include one spoon of matcha powder as you guys know.

mucha is one of the most abundant source of antioxidant in this planet and I use dark leafy green as a base for the smoothie. It has a lot of antioxidants and a lot of good anti-inflammatory properties.

It would be nice to have fresh fruit or fresh berries every single day but that is also a luxury, instead I would highly recommend you guys to check out ecliptic Institute whole food powders from iron.

 Eclectic powders are just really simple; they're raw fresh freeze-dried plants and fruits. They source their ingredients from sustainable harvest at the peak potency and then freeze dry in-house. Freeze dried naturally concentrates by removing the water and just leaving the plants nutrients and has the same balance found in nature.

 So I would highly recommend you guys to go for the powder version from eclectic Institute, I just love it so much. if you want a dash of sweetness reach for a dark cocoa or cacao powder. The Vita's cacao powder is definitely amazing and incorporating in your smoothie or in your breakfast. All you need is some ice cubes that blend everything and you will have this amazing powerful anti-aging smoothie.

CHAPTER TWO

LET'S TALK ABOUT SKINCARE HABITS

In this chapter we are going to talk about skincare habits to prevent signs of aging. The most fundamental rule here is to do no harm as preserve what you already naturally have. I'm not here to tell you what to apply or what not to apply. These are some habits that I can address, that you should be a little bit more mindful of having.

Number one, never give your skin tends to be dried or dehydrated and it's already a known fact that people with oily skin tend to age a little bit slower than those who do have dry skin. People who do live in a dry climate tend to age quicker than those who live in a humid environment. Always keep your skin bouncy, firm and plump and apply a well hydrating, well nourishing and well moisturizing cram.

 Habit Number two, preserve what you already have. so this goes back to our fundamental rule of doing no harm to the skin. Remember that we are all boards with the most effective skin care. It includes your natural skin barrier, your natural healthy microbiome and the pH level by not fluctuating it or by not aggressively abusing those elements. You are already better off than many other people out there.

 Number three is to never stress in the flame or sensitize the skin. Again, inflammation equals Parle aging so if you ever feel like your skin is constantly sensitize and constantly inflamed there is a high chance that you might be overdoing skincare or using a lot of harsh ingredients to the skin.

Habits number four; reduce physical friction or physical contact with your skin. The more facial muscle that you use, you do form some deep set wrinkles that's why the last lines are there. Those are something that naturally happens but at least with skincare you can start by dropping the towel to dry your face or using cotton pad in a very gentle way.

 Last but not least, protect your skin from the UV. Do wear your sunscreen every single day. In one study, it shows that 90% of the skin aging is caused by UV damage and that is a really scary number among all the environmental stressors out there. UV damage is the most accumulative and most damaging to the skin in multiple different levels.

In this section I'm going to highlight some lifestyle habits we should be mindful of. First of all, we have stress management and of course everyone knows how chronic stress can be. Stress is really detrimental in our skin aging and in forming more acne as well. So managing your stress is actually pretty important when it comes to keeping your skin happy and healthy.

WAYS TO MAINTAIN GLOWING SKIN

1. Utilize a protected, mineral-based sunscreen every day.

A spotless, mineral-based SPF ought to be applied every day, throughout the entire year. "Bright radiation is unequivocally cancer-causing," clarifies board-confirmed dermatologist"If you couldn't care less about malignant growth, think vanity—UV beams are the essential driver of the surface and shading changes of skin maturing." To secure your skin, Waldorf suggests utilizing a mineral-based sunscreen (search for dynamic fixings like zinc oxide or titanium dioxide) that is SPF 30 or higher and applying it as the last advance in your skin health management schedule each day. Since mineral sunscreen is an actual hindrance, it ought to be applied as the last advance before cosmetics: Any skin health management actives you attempt to apply after will not enter.

2. Take a stab at enhancing collagen. The most bountiful protein in your body—and your skin—is collagen, and, sadly, our regular stores of this fundamental protein drain as we age. Collagen supplements are crammed with amino acids, which has been appeared to advance our hair, skin, and nail health.* By ingesting the hydrolyzed collagen peptides, the enhancement is consumed by the body and can uphold the skin's cell recharging measure, animating our cell's fibroblasts (or what makes collagen and elastin in the body), in this way advancing a solid, sparkling, firm complexion.*

3. Shed.

"I'm not suggesting a brutal clean or fabric," clarifies board-ensured dermatologist Nancy Samolitis, M.D., who records peeling as one of her top tips for shining skin. "Light shedding every day, with either a nonirritating corrosive chemical or toner that breaks up dead skin cells on a superficial level,

[will] lead to sparkling skin." How so? Eliminating the external layer of dead skin cells will help smooth skin surface, increment the assimilation pace of your healthy skin items, and light up your appearance.

4. Deal with your gut.

Exploration shows that hidden gut medical problems can show on the skin from multiple points of view, from skin inflammation to dermatitis. large gut wellbeing is nuanced and complex, and it's significant (for in this way, such countless purposes behind) everybody to set aside the effort to figure out how to really focus on and support your own special gut greenery. In any case, with the end goal of this article, here's an overall rule: Anything that will harm your gut (sugar, handled food) may likewise harm your skin. Likewise, see: Here's the reason you ought to mend your gut in the event that you need clear skin.

5. Fuse sound fats into your eating routine.

 "Sound fats like those found in nuts, flaxseed, and avocados can assist with recharging your body's capacity to make solid and solid cell films, [which] can ensure against ecological harm by reestablishing the skin obstruction," Samolitis clarifies. Waldorf concurs, clarifying that "not eating sufficient sound fats can make the skin and hair be dry, and expanding these fats in the eating routine may help in certain skin conditions portrayed by exorbitant dryness." Other solid fat food sources to know for gleaming skin incorporate salmon, chia seeds, olive oil, and entire eggs.

6. Keep your skin micro biome adjusted.

Very much like the gut, a sound, adjusted skin micro biome is fundamental to keeping up solid, adjusted skin. These minute microbes keep skin hydrated and flexible, fend off free extremists, fight off disease, and even secure against destructive UV beams. Hold yours under tight restraints by staying away from unforgiving cleansers and scours, which can strip away the fundamental oils and microorganisms that make up the skin micro biome. On the other side, use skin health management items that are figured explicitly to help the skin micro biome, for example, those that contain pre-and proboscis (here's our rundown of the best items to help a solid skin micro biome).

7. Apply healthy skin items just after washing.

Maybe perhaps the most fundamental segments of solid skin is dampness. Notwithstanding a quality skin health management normal, the circumstance in which you apply your items can influence dampness maintenance. Waldorf's top tip: Take to your skin health management routine following jumping out of the shower. "Applying a cream day by day on face and body subsequent to washing recharges and seals in dampness," she says. "It is greatly improved to keep up great skin than to attempt to make up for lost time after skin is dry, aroused, and awkward."

8. Practice a facial back rub schedule. In addition to the fact that it feels charming, however facial back rub can reduce strain and increment course, accordingly assisting with keeping skin cells sound and helping in lymphatic waste. Focus on a day by day facial gua sha routine or utilize a jade roller. It just requires a couple of moments daily, and the post-facial back rub gleam (civility of previously mentioned expanded flow) will be so awesome.

9. Eat cancer prevention agent rich food varieties.

"The more beautiful, the better," Samolitis says. "My top choices are dim, verdant greens and berries." Indeed, leafy foods are viewed as the best wellsprings of cancer prevention agents. Some cell reinforcement pressed food sources to join into your eating routine incorporate blueberries, kale, spinach, and—reward—dim chocolate.

10. Stay dynamic.

Exercise builds blood stream all through the body, subsequently bringing imperative oxygen, supplements, and minerals to the skin. Main concern: Working out prompts more splendid, better-looking skin.

11. Use nutrient C.

Extraordinary compared to other effective elements for sparkling skin, straightforward, is nutrient C—which deals with all skin types to try and out and light up tone. The exploration to back up these cases is sound and huge: Vitamin C can blur hyper pigmentation, secure against natural aggressors, light up skin tone, and advance collagen and easting creation. Primary concern: It's key for shining skin.

12. Try not to pick your skin.
When in doubt of thumb, when your items are applied, keep your (most probable filthy) hands off of your face. "Picking at the skin—pimples, wounds, or simply bothersome regions—causes deteriorating of the issue and at last can [lead to] contamination and scars," Waldorf says.

13. Stay hydrated.

It is anything but a fantasy: Drinking sufficient water is fundamental for in general skin wellbeing. Remaining satisfactorily hydrated keeps your skin saturated, sound, and, you got it, gleaming. That is also the entirety of the other unlimited advantages of drinking enough H20. While eight (8-ounce) glasses each day is the overall rule, water admission isn't one-size-fits-all, so tune in to what your body needs.

14. Utilize a retinoid or retinol elective.

"Regardless of whether your skin improves over-the-counter retinols or original effectiveness retinoid, this fixing is first spot on my list to advance sound, shining skin," Samolitis says. "To start with, it really fixes DNA harm from the sun and climate and can even be defensive against precancerous skin injuries. Second, it holds the top layer of skin back from developing and looking dull by advancing sped up skin cell turnover."

In the event that you conclude retinols are not for you—for reasons unknown—consider bakuchoil, a characteristic elective that yields similar outcomes.

15. Get ordinary facials.
We know, we know—this isn't generally plausible. In any case, if it's in your spending plan, getting ordinary

facials is probably the most ideal approaches to keep a sound, sparkling look, Samolitis says. Preferably, focus on one facial each month, which falls on schedule with your skin cells' regular recharging cycle.

16. Try not to conceivably bother food sources.

You definitely understand what they are: food sources that are bundled, prepared, and high in sugar, just as dairy. "Abundance sugar, dairy, and handled food sources can cause skin aggravation, prompting rashes and breakouts," Samolitis clarifies. On the off chance that you can just focus on disposing of one of these no-no food varieties, make it handled sugar, as late exploration has affirmed the connection between high-sugar food varieties and skin break out, just as broad head-to-toe irritation.

17. Try not to smoke.

Self-evident in any case, for such countless reasons, worth repeating: Smoking effectsly affects your body from head to toe—skin included. While shine is concerned, "smoking limits the oxygen supply to the skin, expands the development of harming free revolutionaries and builds the danger of some skin malignancies," Waldorf clarifies.

18. Enjoy a face veil.

As we would like to think, face covers shouldn't be viewed as an extravagance—you ought to apply these consistently. To boost gleam, decide on hydrating face veil fixings like hyaluronic corrosive, sodium hyaluronate, and nutrient E.

19. Reinforce your skin hindrance.

Bothersome, flaky, dry skin? Your skin hindrance is likely undermined. Fortify it by utilizing lotions and chemicals that are figured with ceramides, a fundamental segment of the skin obstruction (that can be stripped away by things like over cleansing).

20. Get your magnificence rest.

One more significant motivation to focus on rest: Inadequate or upset rest can unleash destruction on your skin. Examination has shown that helpless rest quality can add to expanded indications of skin maturing (scarce differences and wrinkles) and traded off skin boundary work. Similarly as with water, eight hours is the standard dependable guideline for rest, however consistently tune in to your body.

21. Take nicotinamide riboside.

In fact called nicotinamide riboside (NR), this atom attempts to fix and reestablish cell wellbeing and capacity—inside and out. In the body, this type of nutrient B3 is transformed into the coenzyme NAD. Like most other beneficial things (collagen, elastin, hyaluronic corrosive—and so on), our degrees of NAD+ normally decay with age, so supplanting what gets lost offers a large group of benefits.

mindbodygreen's nr+ is clinically demonstrated enhancement to expand levels of NAD+. Plus it works in a horde of extra approaches to help solid, gleaming skin: specifically, giving cancer prevention agent security, reestablishing skin hindrance work, and recharging ceramide levels.*

22. Keep your cosmetics—and cosmetics devices—clean.

Cosmetics brushes, packs, and wipes are fundamentally favorable places for the expansion of microorganisms, dead skin cells, oil, and grime—all of which can genuinely thwart your journey for shining skin. In this way, keep things sterile! Clean your cosmetics apparatuses consistently, in a perfect world each and every other week.

23. Keep things tepid.

Quite possibly the most well-known face-washing botches: utilizing some unacceptable water temperature. Flushing your appearance (and hair) with water that is too hot can strip your skin boundary of its normal oils, which can dry out the skin and lead to an undermined obstruction. Too-cool water will not take care of business and might leave earth and cosmetics on your skin. So with regards to purifying, stick to water temperatures that are tepid.

24. Limit pressure.

More difficult than one might expect, we know, however sensations of ongoing pressure can truly harm your skin—and surprisingly trigger a large group of issues, including dermatitis and psoriasis. Even more motivation to focus on a legitimate self-care normal, whatever that may look like for you (despite the fact that may we propose a couple previously mentioned tips like setting aside a few minutes for face veils, facials, exercise, and magnificence rest).

25. Saturate.

Need we say more? Keeping skin saturated is probably the speediest pass to a sparkling composition. Try not to hold back on every day lotion, regardless of whether you have normally slick skin, and put resources into fixings that are demonstrated to hydrate (like peptides, electrolytes, and ceramides).

CHAPTER THREE

EXERCISING HABIT

The Perfect Weekly Workout Routine

The primary inquiry on numerous individuals' brains when they're thinking about beginning an activity schedule:

How frequently would it be a good idea for you to work out? Furthermore, what would it be advisable for you to do during every exercise to make the most out of it?

Like most things in the wellness world, nobody answers that question: It all relies upon your wellness foundation, the time you have accessible, and your own objectives. The best exercise routine for you—and how long you work out—might appear to be quite unique from a strong daily practice for another person. It's not super-supportive, for example, to demonstrate your week after week exercise routine after somebody prepared to run a long-distance race in case you're keen on figuring out how to strength train.

In any case, if you don't have super-explicit wellness objectives—say, you're searching for a cycle of everything to expand strength and perseverance so you can move better and feel good—there are a few rules that can help you sort out a feasible exercise program. Here, what you need to think about how frequently you should function out, what to zero in on, and how to make it a propensity that sticks.

How frequently would it be a good idea for you to work out every week?

As we said, there's no basic recipe that is appropriate for everybody. In case you're looking to amp up your wellness level, your sorcery number of days relies upon how dynamic you as of now are.

For instance, you'll presumably see physical (and mental) results from one day seven days if you don't But in case you're utilized to different exercise days seven days, one day likely will not move your body enough to keep up your wellness or gain ground.

The breakdown differs depending upon your particular objectives, yet by and large, four to five days seven days will get the job done if you're meaning to improve or keep up your wellness.

Obviously, in case you're simply beginning and don't practice at present, that may be too large of a seize first, says ACE-affirmed mentor Sivan Fagan, proprietor of Strong with Sivan in Baltimore. Furthermore, that can divert you off totally from working out. All things considered, have a go at the beginning with two exercises every week, which you can increment continuously.

How do you construct functioning out into a propensity?

Defining a feasible objective for how frequently you'll begin functioning out every week can be useful by ensuring you don't get worn out.

In any case, going for a touch of development every day, regardless of whether you're not doing a real exercise, can likewise help you make working out a propensity that will stick, she says. This may mean a 10-minute walk or a progression of delicate stretches.

Another significant thought is deciding when you'll work out. Once more, there's no correct response to this, yet it assists with investigating your timetable when sorting out when you should pencil in your exercise. For example, if your mornings are super-furious with heaps of a minute ago a change, it very well may act naturally crush to anticipate morning exercises, says Fagan. Around there, an evening or evening exercise might be bound to occur as planned.

Also, focus on your body as well: Some individuals feel more invigorated in the first part of the day, while others are hauling. Coordinating up your exercise time to when you feel the best can make you bound to need to stay with it

What should every day of working out resemble?

If you need to work out five days of the week and are chipping away at both strength and cardiovascular wellness, attempt three days of solidarity preparing, two days of cardio, and two days of dynamic rest. If you need to work out four days per week, consider your objectives: If you need to add muscle, cut a cardio day. On the off chance that you need to improve perseverance, avoid a strength day. Or on the other hand, switch it every week.

WATCH

Keep in mind that it's essential to be sensible about your own timetable when you're asking yourself what number of times each week would be a good idea for me to work out? If four days works better for you than five days, just stick to it. Be that as it may if five days is sensible, amazing!

In any case, here's the way (and when and why) to squash it at everyone.

Strength Training: 2–3 Times Each Week

Why: Strength preparing is a very significant approach to keep your body uses for the long stretch, says Fagan: It forestalls the bone misfortune and muscle misfortune that accompanies maturing. It additionally reinforces your joints as well.

How: To assemble bulk, you should attempt to work for each muscle bunch a few times each week. So in a multi-day strength plan, this implies you should expect to do full-body exercises—you'll need to hit the significant muscle gatherings of your upper and lower body. That may seem as though a ton, however, that is the place where compound activities come in. Moves like squats lurches, columns, and chest squeeze work more than each muscle bunch in turn, so you get all the more value for your money.

You likewise need to have harmony between pushing developments (like an overhead press or chest press) and pulling developments (like with a column). Keep in mind, strength preparation isn't just about freeloads or machines—dominating bodyweight moves will challenge your muscles as well.

Go for 12-15 reps for each set when you are simply beginning. Whenever you've gotten more OK with the moves, you can diminish the reps as you add more weight. One to two arrangements of each activity is sufficient for your first month, after which you might need to expand it to three.

You ought to do various moves in every one of the three strength meetings, however, rehash those equivalent moves each week.

I would remain with a program for about a month and a half and logically increase the weight.

[The week before your last week] I would have a tad of a drop-off to give your body a tad of recuperation, and the most recent week, truly push it hard.

How Long: A strength-instructional course should last 40 to an hour, in addition to froth rolling and a speedy warm-up in advance.

Cardio: 2–3 Times Each Week

Why: As significant for what it's worth to strength train, cardio has its place in a fair exercise routine as well. "Doing cardio keeps your circulatory framework working ideally, assisting you with recuperating quicker... [And it] keeps your perseverance up. "It likewise builds your VO2 max, which assists your body with using oxygen."

How: You have a huge load of alternatives: an open-air run, a bicycle ride, past curved machine if your rec center is open and you feel good going—the rundown goes on. Utilitarian developments, as portable weight swings, and readiness work can likewise consider cardio, insofar as you're doing what's needed reps during a specific time span to keep your pulse raised.

"Regardless of whether something is cardiovascular relies upon where your pulse is at and how long you're doing it for," Target pulses are diverse for everybody, I would recommend that a decent pattern to target during your cardio schedules is somewhere in the range of 120 and 150 beats each moment for 45 to an hour.

Another choice is span preparing, where you buckle down for a short measure of time and substitute that with recuperation periods. You can do this with essentially anything—indoor line machine, bicycle, running, utilitarian developments, and so on.

5 Types of Vitafusion Gummy Vitamins Were Just Recalled Because They May Contain Metal

A 30-Minute Full-Body Workout That Really Works Your Abs

There are likewise a lot of cardio classes out there that you can attempt essentially (a significant number of which will work your muscles all in all too).

How Long: The American College of Sports Medicine prescribes logging 150 minutes of moderate-to-serious action each week. How you split that up will rely upon what sort of preparing you're doing (longer, consistent state meetings versus more limited HIIT exercises).

Rest Days: 2 Times Each Week

Why: Taking a break allows your body to recuperate and revamp so you can return to your exercises revived and prepared to shake it. A rest day ought to really be viewed as dynamic recuperation, which means you don't need to head out to the rec center or break genuine perspiration, yet you ought to accomplish something.

"It's not just about the actual recuperation—it's additionally the psychological, "Accomplishing something that you make the most of that is dynamic is extraordinary for the brain... and it aids remaining weakness." Plus, it keeps up your molding.

How: Whether you do some extending or simply go for a stroll, dynamic recuperation shouldn't need a huge load of exertion like an exercise day, however it ought to make your move. You can likewise attempt a virtual remedial class, as delicate yoga or a casual tangle Pilates class.

Where you place these rest days is dependent upon you—in the event that you do your exercises Monday through Friday, don't hesitate to require the entire end of the week off Or you could split them up by doing a strength day, a cardio day, at that point a rest day prior to returning to weight preparing. Albeit the request doesn't actually matter, I suggest not dealing with strength two days straight. You need to give your body 48 hours to recuperate.

How Long: Aim for 30 minutes or an hour of active recuperation.

CHAPTER FOUR

LOOK INTO YOUR SLEEPING HABIT

Next we're gonna look into your sleeping habit. First of all, if you are a side sleeper it's time to switch to a back sleeper. It does make a huge difference. Also, consider switching your pillowcase from cotton to silk because it really does make a difference. Sick pillowcases are better at temperature regulation and it's more hygienic and gives you less wrinkles.

Sleep deprivation does affect your skin to age more. it was found that poor quality sleep tend to show more signs of aging way quicker than those who do get regular hours of sleep such as seven to eight hours.

They also recover much slower after skin barrier disruption.

 Next is exercise. You don't need to do any hardcore or high-intensity workout every single day. if that's your thing don't go for it but if you have not exercised before definitely start with something that is low-impact that is mild but just do it consistently in a regular basis because by working out ,it does increase your blood circulation.

 It will invite more oxygen to flow within the body which eventually makes your body to absorb more nutrients from the food that you take and from the supplements that you take. So definitely, a really big thing is affecting your overall health and your skin's health in general.

17 TIPS TO SLEEP BETTER AT NIGHT

1. Increment brilliant light openness during the day

Your body makes some normal memories keeping clock known as your circadian It influences your mind, body, and chemicals, assisting you with remaining conscious and advising your body when it's an ideal opportunity to rest

Brilliant light during the day helps keep your cadence strong. It improves daytime energy, just as evening time rest quality and length in individuals with a sleeping disorder, daytime splendid light openness improved rest quality and term. It additionally decreased the time it took to nod off by 83% A comparative report in more established grown-ups tracked down that 2 hours of brilliant light openness during the day expanded the measure of rest by 2 hours and rest productivity by 80% While most exploration includes individuals with serious rest issues, day by day light openness will help you whether you experience normal rest or not.

Take a stab at getting every day daylight openness or — if this isn't viable — put resources into a counterfeit splendid light gadget or bulbs.

Every day daylight or fake brilliant light can improve rest quality and term, particularly on the off chance that you have serious rest issues or a sleeping disorder.

2. Lessen blue light openness in the evening

Openness to light during the day is valuable, yet evening time light openness has the contrary impact Again, this is because of its impact on your circadian beat, fooling your mind into believing it's still daytime. This lessens chemicals like melatonin, which assist you with unwinding and get profound rest

Blue light — which electronic gadgets like cell phones and PCs produce in enormous sums — is the most exceedingly terrible in such manner.

- **There are a few mainstream** techniques you can use to decrease evening blue light openness these include:

- **Wear glasses that square blue light** download an application, for example, f.lux to obstruct blue light on your PC or PC.

- **Install an application that squares blue** light on your cell phone. The application is available for all kinds of phones

- **Stop sitting in front of the TV and mood killer any brilliant lights 2 hours prior to going to bed.**

Blue light fools your body into speculation it's daytime. There are a few different ways you can diminish blue light openness in the evening.

3. Avoid late night caffeine consumption

Caffeine has lots benefit for the body and is devoured by more than half of the Americas population.

A solitary portion can improve center, energy, and sports execution

Be that as it may, when burned-through late in the day, caffeine invigorates your sensory system and may prevent your body from normally unwinding around evening time.

In one examination, burning-through caffeine as long as 6 hours before bed altogether demolished rest quality Caffeine can remain raised in your blood for 6–8 hours isn't suggested, particularly in case you're delicate to caffeine or experience difficulty dozing If you do hunger for some espresso in the late evening or evening, stay with decaffeinated espresso.

Caffeine can altogether deteriorate rest quality, particularly on the off chance that you drink huge sums in the late evening or evening.

4. Decrease unpredictable or long daytime snoozes

While short force snoozes are valuable, long or unpredictable resting during the day can contrarily influence your rest.

Dozing in the daytime can befuddle your inner clock, implying that you may battle to rest around evening time truth be told, in one examination, members wound up being sleepier during the day subsequent to taking daytime snoozes

Another examination noticed that while snoozing for 30 minutes or less can upgrade daytime cerebrum work, longer rests can hurt well-being and rest quality However, a few investigations show that the individuals who are accustomed to taking customary daytime rest don't encounter helpless rest quality or disturbed rest around evening time.

On the off chance that you take ordinary daytime snoozes and rest soundly, you shouldn't stress. The impacts of resting rely upon the person

Long daytime rests may debilitate rest quality. In the event that you experience difficulty resting around evening time, quit snoozing or abbreviate your snoozes.

5. Attempt to rest and wake at reliable occasions

Your body's circadian cadence capacities on a set circle, adjusting itself to dawn and dusk.

Being reliable with your rest and waking occasions can help long haul rest quality

One investigation noticed that members who had sporadic dozing designs and hit the hay late on the ends of the week revealed helpless rest (Other examinations have featured that unpredictable rest examples can modify your circadian musicality and levels of melatonin, which signal your mind to rest If you battle with rest, attempt to start awakening and hitting the hay at comparable occasions. Following a little while, you may not need caution.

Attempt to get into an ordinary rest/wake cycle — particularly at the ends of the week. On the off chance that conceivable, attempt to awaken normally at a comparative time each day.

6. Take a melatonin supplement

Melatonin is a key rest chemical that advises your cerebrum when it's an ideal opportunity to unwind and make a beeline for bed

Melatonin supplements are an incredibly mainstream tranquilizer.

Regularly used to treat sleep deprivation, melatonin might be perhaps the simplest approach to In one examination, taking 2 mg of melatonin before bed improved rest quality and energy the following day and assisted individuals with nodding off quicker.

In another examination, half of the gathering nodded off quicker and had a 15% improvement in rest quality

Also, no withdrawal impacts were accounted for in both of the above investigations.

Melatonin is likewise valuable when heading out and acclimating to another time region, as it helps your body's circadian musicality recover to business as usual

Start with a low portion to evaluate your resistance and afterward increment it gradually on a case-by-case basis. Since melatonin may adjust mind science, it's exhorted that you check with a medical services supplier before use.

You ought to likewise talk with them in case you're considering utilizing melatonin as a tranquilizer for your youngster, as long haul utilization of this enhancement in kids has not been very much examined.

A melatonin supplement is a simple method to improve rest quality and nod off quicker. Take 1–5 mg around 30–an hour prior to making a beeline for bed.

7. Think about these different enhancements

A few enhancements can incite unwinding and help you rest, including:

- Ginkgo biloba: A characteristic spice with numerous advantages, it might help rest, unwinding, and stress decrease, however, the proof is restricted. Take 250 mg 30–an hour prior to bed Glycine: A couple of studies show that taking 3 grams of the amino corrosive glycine can improve rest quality Valerian root: Several investigations propose that valerian can help you nod off and improve rest quality. Take 500 mg before bed. Magnesium can improve unwinding and upgrade rest quality (L-theanine: An amino corrosive, L-theanine can improve unwinding and rest. Take 100–200 mg before bed Lavender: An incredible spice with numerous medical advantages, lavender can incite a quieting and stationary impact to improve rest. Take 80–160 mg containing 25–46% linalool

Try to just attempt these enhancements each in turn. While they're not an enchantment slug for rest issues, they can be helpful when joined with other regular dozing techniques.

A few enhancements, including lavender and magnesium, can assist with unwinding and rest quality when joined with different techniques.

8. Try not to drink liquor

Two or three beverages around evening time can adversely influence your rest and chemicals.

Liquor is known to cause or expand the indications of rest apnea, wheezing, and disturbed rest designs It additionally changes evening melatonin creation, which assumes a vital part in your body's circadian mood, Another investigation found that liquor utilization around evening time diminished the regular evening rises in human development chemical (HGH), which assumes a part in your circadian musicality and has numerous other key capacities

Keep away from liquor before bed, as it can lessen evening melatonin creation and lead to upset rest designs.

9. Improve your room climate

Numerous individuals accept that the room climate and its arrangement are key factors in getting a decent night's rest.

These variables incorporate temperature, clamor, outer lights, and furniture game plan numerous investigations bring up that outside commotion, regularly from traffic, can cause helpless rest and long haul medical problems in a single report on the room climate of ladies, around half of the members saw improved rest quality when commotion and light lessened

To enhance your room climate, attempt to limit outer commotion, light, and counterfeit lights from gadgets like morning timers. Ensure your room is a calm, unwinding, clean, and pleasant spot.

Upgrade your room climate by disposing of outside light and commotion to improve rest.

10. Set your room temperature

Body and room temperature can likewise significantly influence rest quality.

As you may have encountered throughout the mid-year or in hot areas, it tends to be extremely difficult to get a decent night's rest when it's excessively warm.

One investigation found that room temperature influenced rest quality more than outer commotion Other examinations uncover that expanded body and room temperature can diminish rest quality and increment alertness

Around 70°F is by all accounts an agreeable temperature for the vast majority, in spite of the fact that it relies upon your inclinations and propensities.

Test various temperatures to discover which is generally agreeable for you. Around 70°F (20°C) is best for a great many people.

11. Try not to eat late in the evening

Eating late around evening time may contrarily influence both rest quality and the common arrival of HGH and melatonin

All things considered, the quality and sort of your late-night tidbit may assume a part too.

In one investigation, a high carb supper was eaten 4 hours before bed assisted individuals with nodding off

Curiously, one examination found that a low carb diet likewise improved rest, demonstrating that carbs aren't generally fundamental, particularly in case you're utilized to a low carb diet

Burning-through an enormous supper before bed can prompt helpless rest and chemical interruption. Notwithstanding, certain dinners and snacks a couple of hours before bed may help.

16. Exercise routinely — however not before bed

Exercise is extraordinary compared to other science-supported approaches to improve your rest and wellbeing.

It can upgrade all parts of rest and has been utilized to diminish manifestations of sleep deprivation (One investigation in more seasoned grown-ups confirmed that activity almost divided the measure of time it took to nod off and gave 41 additional minutes of rest around evening time In individuals with serious sleep deprivation, practice offered a larger number of advantages than most medications. Exercise diminished chance to nod off by 55%, all out night attentiveness by 30%, and tension by 15% while expanding absolute rest time by 18% Although day by day practice is key for a decent night's rest, performing it past the point of no return in the day may mess rest up.

This is because of the stimulatory impact of activity, which expands readiness and chemicals like epinephrine and adrenaline.

Notwithstanding, a few examinations show no adverse consequences, so it obviously relies upon the person

Standard exercise during sunlight hours is probably the most ideal approaches to guarantee a decent night's rest.

17. Try not to drink any fluids before bed

Nocturia is the clinical term for unnecessary pee during the evening. It influences rest quality and daytime energy

Drinking a lot of fluids before bed can prompt comparative side effects, however a few group are more delicate than others.

Despite the fact that hydration is fundamental for your wellbeing, it's astute to decrease your liquid admission in the late evening.

Attempt to not drink any liquids 1–2 hours prior to heading to sleep.

You ought to likewise utilize the restroom just prior to heading to sleep, as this may diminish your odds of waking in the evening.

Lessen liquid admission in the late evening and attempt to utilize the washroom just before bed.

CHAPTER FIVE

CONCLUSION

I encourage you to apply everything you have read in this book and your life will definitely not remain the same.